Bernhard Johannes Schmidt

The Munchausen Syndrome by Proxy as a Group Phenomenon

Contributions to Clinical Social Psychology

Contributions to Clinical Social Psychology
No. 7

Bernhard J. Schmidt

The
Munchausen Syndrome by Proxy
as a Group Phenomenon

ISBN: 978-83752624670

Manufacture and Publisher:
BoD – Books on Demand, Norderstedt, Germany

Bibliographic information from the German National Library:
The German National Library lists this publication in the
Deutschen Nationalbibliografie (German National Bibliography;
detailed bibliographic data can be found on the internet at
http://dnb.dnb.de.)

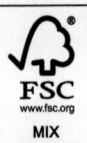

Table of content

I.   Introduction...9

II.   Munchausen Syndrome by proxy.................11

   1 MSbP – Basics.....................................13

      1.1 Motivations...................................15

      1.2 Denial of responsibility..............17

III.   Group phenomena.......................................20

   1 Group properties in general.............................20

   2 Advantages of groups.....................................21

      2.1 Duration of existence..................21

      2.2 Influence / advocacy...................22

      2.3 The relationship changes............22

      2.4 Protection of the individual........22

      2.5 Not in the secret........................23

      2.6 Not just against experts.............23

   3 Negative characteristics of groups...................23

      3.1 High pressure to conform..........24

      3.2 One-sided information................25

      3.3 Falsification of information........25

      3.4 Experts without expertise..........25

      3.5 Mixing of interests....................26

      3.6 Proselytizing.............................27

   4 Groups with pathological targets....................28

IV. MSbP as a group phenomenon......................29

   1 Vulnerability ./. illness.............................31

   2 Autism - the made-up disease........................32

   3 Origin of the dogma system..........................34

V. Excursus: The power of the organization......37

VI. MSbP in autism "theory" and "therapy"......39

   1 Denial of responsibility....................................39

   2 Chronic illness..40

   3 Immunization and discrediting........................41

   4 Funding and ignoring...42

     4.1 Ignoring alternative theories and therapies
....43

   5 Separation...44

   6 Lack of valid diagnosis....................................44

VII. Forms of ill-treatment.................................46

   1 Omission..47

   2 Biochemical "interventions"............................49

     2.1 DAN! as an example of biochemical "thera-
pies"..50

   3 "Behavioral Therapies"....................................54

     3.1 ABA...55

     3.2 TEACCH..59

VIII. The MSbP system.......................................61

IX. Parents as organized groups........................63

1   Parents' motivations...66

   1.1   Healthy motivation - help for the child.....67

   1.2   Morbid motivations.....................................67

2   Autismus Deutschland e.V. as an an example..68

   2.1   Striving for attention..................................69

   2.2   Pretend Help...69

   2.3   Preventing effective aid.............................70

   2.4   Suppression and discrediting of helpful information..70

X. Doctors / psychologists as (co-) perpetrators 72

1   Psychological primitivism...............................72

   1.1   Behaviorism...73

   1.2   Static instead of dynamic development.....73

   1.3   Isolated instead of social psychological....74

   1.4   Hindsight-bias on diagnosis.......................74

2   Lack of professional distance..........................75

3   Induced disease..78

   3.1   No valid diagnosis.....................................81

   3.2   Disease-inducing "therapies"....................85

      3.2.a   ABA and derivatives.........................87

      3.2.b   PECS...89

      3.2.c   Floortime (DIR)................................90

4   Effects...91

XI. Autistic self-advocates..................................92

    1 Motivations...92

    2 Have a stabilizing effect...................................92

    3 Prevent "abuse through treatment"..................93

    4 Promote "abuse through omission".................93

XII. Summary...94

    1 Need for clinical social psychology................94

XIII. Appendix: Autism as Vulnerability...........96

    Bibliography..100

I. INTRODUCTION

The aim of this book is twofold.

First, as part of the series "Contributions to clinical social psychology", the importance and necessity of clinical social psychology should be shown.

Both through the spread of mass media since the beginning of the 20th century as a form of one-sided influence, and through the emergence of social media in the last few decades as a form of mutual influence, diverse new possibilities arise.

On the one hand, there are possibilities for realizing pathological group processes, of which the propaganda of the Nazi regime is an example,

on the other hand, there is also the possibility of recognizing such processes. This also enables the perception and analysis of further connections between mental disorders as well as (stabilizing) interactions between various groups.

It will also be shown that as soon as one overcomes the "individualization of the irrational" (Schmidt; Ganz 2017) through the perspective of clinical social psychology, the frequency of personality disorders and associated syndromes such as the Munchausen syndrome by proxy must also be reassessed.

The change of perspectives, from "frames of reference" (West 1981, Schmidt 2018), always harbors the danger that the application will be exaggerated, as many examples in the history of science show.

The second aim is therefore to prevent misuse of the following statements from the outset.

It is not the aim of this book to deny autism or the suffering of many autistic people – on the contrary. By presenting the 'Munchausen syndrome by proxy as a group phenomenon' using the example of autism, it is intended to show how this syndrome, via the organization in self-help groups, has led to autistic people being denied effective help and therapies for half a century . And that instead these people were and still are mistreated with absurd "therapies". So please do not refer to this book if you want to portray autism in general as if autism was invented by parents with Munchausen proxy syndrome.

II. MUNCHAUSEN SYNDROME BY PROXY

The syndrome appears in the specialist literature under various names:

- 'Fabricated or Induced Illness by Carers' (FII) [Davis et al. 2019]

- Meadow's syndrome
  [Warner 1984], named after Roy Meadow [1977]

- Factitious Disorder by Proxy (FDP)
"Whereas "Munchausen by proxy" (or "Munchausen syndrome by proxy") is the better known term for the phenomenon, "factitious disorder by proxy" and "facti-tious disorder imposed on another" are diagnostic terms being considered for the upcoming edition of the Diagno-stic and Statistical Manual of Mental Disorders (DSM-5; Dimsdale et al. 2009)." [Frye; Feldman 2011]

- Munchausen Syndrome by Proxy (MSbP)

All of these terms contain slightly different accents, but at the same time describe the same syndrome.

However, a critical examination of the question of who and what should be the focus of both the definition and the consideration should not be overlooked: the motivations of the primary caregiver as the perpetrator, or the consequences for the maltreated child.

"The varied terminology currently used reflects uncertainty as to whether the definition should focus on parental behaviour or motivation, or on the harm to the child. The latter position has been advocated by both RCPCH and the American Academy of Paediatrics 'to reflect emphasis on the child as the victim... rather than on the mental status or motivation of the caregiver who has caused the signs and/or symptoms'." [Davis et al. 2019]

In the following, the different terms will appear in quotations, but otherwise the abbreviation MSbP for Munchausen Syndrome by Proxy is used. And even if the mother or other primary caregiver who harm the child are in part certainly victims themselves, they will be referred to as "perpetrators" in the following. This is mainly because of the focus on the child and his abuse.

1   MSbP – Basics

An excerpt from Frye and Feldman should serve as a definition:

"Factitious disorder by proxy (FDP), historically known as Munchausen syndrome by proxy, is a diagnosis applied to parents and other caregivers who intentionally feign, exaggerate, and/or induce illness or injury in a child to get attention from health professionals and others." [Frye; Feldman 2011]

The MSbP / FDP does not only appear in the clinical area, but also in the educational and school area.

"A review of the recent literature and our experience as consultants indicate clearly that FDP has emerged in educational settings as well. Variants of educational FDP include parents of children with real or fabricated physical disabilities who request excessive or unneeded school health services and parents who request extensive education-related evaluations for children who do not demonstrate any educational need." [Frye; Feldman 2011]

And there are not only physical but also mental disorders as a means to the MSbP end, as well as a combination:

"Neurological and neuropsychiatric presentations including learning difficulty and developmental delay are represented briefly in the literature." [Davis et al. 2019]

and

"DSM-IV-Text Revision (DSM-IV-TR; American Psychiatric Association 2000) includes criteria for factitious disorder that specify three different subtypes—the first with primarily physical symptoms, the second with primarily psychological symptoms, and the third with both psychological and physical symptoms. FDP is included within the residual category of 'factitious disorder not otherwise specified.'" [Frye; Feldman 2011]

The perpetrator is mainly the child's mother, who sees herself as an "expert", but other primary caregivers can also be involved or responsible.

"FII inevitably involves the carer and the child. We use 'carer' to include any primary caregiver. Most cases involve mothers. Fathers or male carers are seldom solely

14

involved. They may collude with or be sidelined by the 'expert' mother." [Davis et al. 2019]

The perpetrators usually come from a medical / psychological environment or have acquired the relevant knowledge.

1.1   Motivations

Even if the question of the perpetrators' motivations should not be in the foreground, these are important for understanding the syndrome.

"There are two different starting points or carer motivations, which are necessary but not sufficient for FII to occur. Both are underpinned by the carer's need for their child to be recognised and treated as ill or more ill or disabled than the child is:
1. In the first, the child is being used to fulfil the carer's needs and gains.
Rarely the carer shows a callous disregard for the child's suffering.
There are different reasons underpinning the carer's needs. They include:

— Fulfilment of the carer's unmet emotional needs for attention and status, for example in personality disorder.*

— Financial or material gain (eg, disability or carer benefits).*

— Deflecting blame from the carer for parenting difficulties or a child's behavioural problems.

— Maintaining closeness to child.

— Negativity towards/disappointment with the child 'justified' by evidence of disorder in the child.

*More likely to include deception.

2. The second includes a carer's erroneous beliefs, extreme anxiety and concern about the child's state of health, to the detriment of the child. Rarely, these beliefs are delusional or may be associated with a carer's autism spectrum disorder. These motivations rarely lead to deceptive carer behaviour." [Davis et al. 2019]

With all "understanding" of the needs of the perpetrators, however, it must not be overlooked that these lead to massive forms of abuse and mistreatment of the child.

"The MSbP is a special form of the violence – a parent to gain the attention and compassion of the surrounding is able to make a physical and emotional harm to a child. There also appears the threat of child's life, hospitalizati-

on and more over potentially harmful medical activities, not only to healthy children, but also chronically ill." [Majda et al. 2019]

In doing so, the offender or offenders sometimes also give the child various dangerous to life-threatening "treatments" in order to gain attention for themselves.

"Usually recognized as a form of child maltreatment, the typical motivation for a parent to harm a child in this way is to assume the "sick role" vicariously and get attention and nurturance for being a longsuffering parent of a chronically ill child." [Frye; Feldman 2011]

1.2   Denial of responsibility

The basic problem of mental disorders is well known that they often lack insight into the disease.
So it is not surprising that the perpetrators of MSbP are hardly aware of any guilt, and often even dismiss it far from themselves. On the contrary, as will be shown, the suppression of (co-) responsibility can be the cause of the formation of an MSbP in the first place.

"Only rarely have mothers readily acknowledged their role in MSBP, though some degree of admission may be

likelier in cases in which the alleged abuse is compara-
tively mild. Eventually, sometimes years after initial con-
frontation, they make indirect admissions with statements
such as, ‚I guess I had a nervous breakdown'. In many
cases, the parent does not appear to be consciously lying
while offering the denial. Instead, her thinking may best
be characterized as ‚quasi-delusional'; that is, while
lacking a formal thought disorder, she may come to belie-
ve, at least intermittently, that her child has a primary,
not induced, illness. In scattered cases, mothers will ad-
mit that they must have harmed their children based
upon the compelling evidence but that they have no re-
collection of having behaved in this way; these individu-
als may have had episodes of authentic dissociation.
Other mothers will claim to have induced illness in the
child ‚just this one time', allegedly intending only that
the staff heighten its vigilance to the child's medical sta-
tus; in these situations, the mother denies neither the evi-
dence nor her culpability, but instead minimizes the
seriousness of the possible consequences of the abuse."
[Feldman 1994]

The denial of responsibility is systematically strength-
ened. On the one hand through the false self-perception
as an expert, and on the other hand through the successful
deception of medical or psychological staff. With the

consent of doctors and psychologists, the perpetrator is encouraged in his own behavior.

The successful deception of doctors and psychologists as well as of themselves reinforce each other.

The more successful the self-deception with regard to the damage to the child and the motives behind it, the easier it is to deceive doctors and psychologists ... whereby a greater degree of security in self-deception and deception is achieved.

If one wanted to assign the MSbP to a personality disorder, then the narcissistic personality disorder would offer itself. The need for attention and self-affirmation, the lack of a sense of injustice, and the frequently occurring mythomania that manifests itself through inventing or exaggerating diseases, all indicate that this personality disorder underlies the MSbP.

In addition, there is the refusal and inability to perceive reality in general, and thus also differences in competence, combined with the need for effectiveness.

See also Schmidt, B.; Ganz, A. (2017) „*Symbiotischer Narzissmus als Gruppenphänomen*".

III. GROUP PHENOMENA

To understand MSbP as a group phenomenon, in addition to knowledge of the basics of MSbP, it is also necessary to consider the characteristics of groups.

1   Group properties in general

Groups in their various forms and with the most varied of characteristics determine our coexistence. Only the hermit exists - at least largely - without group activities. Groups enable individuals to realize their interests and goals in association with others.

Even if we do not necessarily perceive ourselves that way, humans are not a "we-less I" (Norbert Elias), but a "pack animal".

From the family as a core group to long-term care and death insurance, people depend on belonging to different groups.

Groups come in all sorts of ways, with different goals, both as secret societies and as public organizations. The different needs and interests of people are reflected in appropriate groups.

The complexity of the influences and interactions between individuals and groups are, among other things,

competently and extensively presented in M. Wetherell (1996).
The properties of groups that are relevant to the topic are only briefly addressed here.

2 Advantages of groups

The group offers the individual a number of, often indispensable, advantages. Yes, without groups and group membership people could not live and survive at all.
By belonging to a group, identity is generated, behavior is determined, culture and language are developed and passed on ...

2.1 Duration of existence

Behaviors and norms are developed, preserved and handed down within groups. Without groups, the experiences and discoveries made by the individual would be lost with death.
Groups ensure the "survival" of knowledge and traditions beyond death. An example of group longevity is the Catholic Church.

2.2   Influence / advocacy

However, groups not only have an internal effect, i.e. between the group as such and its members as individuals, but often also an external effect.

The individual can only represent his interests efficiently through the group.

2.3   The relationship changes

By belonging to a group, people are no longer opposed to a group as an individual, be it another group at the same level or an authority, government etc.

He acts as part of a group, with the support and protection of this group, against other groups.

2.4   Protection of the individual

The group offers the individual protection against other individuals, but above all against other groups.

2.5 Not in the secret

As an individual, you rarely get public attention. However, as the group grows, so does public awareness. Conversely, the size of the group often increases with the public media perception.

2.6 Not just against experts

By belonging to a group, the individual is no longer subordinate to the experts. The group becomes a "meta-expert" whose expertise the member participates in. As a member, it becomes a quasi-expert itself. See also Charles K. West (1981) „*The social and psychological distortion of information.*"

3 Negative characteristics of groups

People live in a constant tension between "I" and "we", between individuality and group membership.
These tensions and attempts to master them are exemplified on the one hand in direct and indirect compulsory membership. And on the other hand, based on the high hurdles for exclusion from the party.

With the compulsory membership one can differentiate between those with which membership

- is compulsory in a certain group
- it is mandatory, but the choice remains free
- voluntary, but limited to a group as there are no alternatives.

If measure and center are lost in this tense relationship, if there is a pronounced one-sidedness, then negative characteristics are the result.

And when the normal conflict between the various interests, views and beliefs represented by groups escalates, negative consequences result. The Inquisition is an example of this.

3.1 High pressure to conform

The creation and existence of groups presupposes conformity and also a certain pressure to conform. The required conformity can be based on a common interest, e.g. the breeding of ornamental fish. Within this common interest, however, a free exchange of information is sought. At the other end of the scale are groups that demand compliance with a strict dogma. These can be found among others in extreme political positions, world views ...

In his publications on "Group think", Irving Janis described the devastating consequences that pressure to conform within groups can have.

3.2   One-sided information

The group members only receive information that complies with the group objectives. The individual "confirmation bias" is institutionalized - be it consciously or unconsciously.
Information that contradicts the group's opinion is either suppressed or discredited, for example, as "fake news". So arise „communities of ignorance" (Schmidt 2019).

3.3   Falsification of information

In order to consolidate and justify the group positions, information is consciously or unconsciously falsified or faked. The individual "self-serving bias" is being expanded and institutionalized.

3.4   Experts without expertise

Pseudo-experts emerge whose competence is presumed based on their group membership, but is not available. Missing expertise is replaced by group membership and a corresponding status within the group. See also Charles K. West (1981).

3.5   Mixing of interests

At a large German automobile club, the interests of most members are probably the included breakdown assistance, monetary benefits, etc.

And yet this club also represents very influential and extensive political and commercial positions that are not necessarily shared by all members.

With the size of a group, the influence of the individual member on the group also decreases, which is why there is hardly anything to counteract such developments.

The intermingling of interests is particularly great when it is alleged that the interests of others rather than one's own are to be asserted, as has been the case for decades with development aid. Here, as with assistance for the disabled, one often finds paternalistic tutelage that largely hides various personal interests. Groups that supposedly represent the interests of others should always be viewed with skepticism.

3.6 Proselytizing

Only a few groups have an urge to proselytize. This is usually based on a dogmatism as group content, in connection with an ideologization as an "exclusive promise of salvation" (Schmidt; Ganz 2017). The aim of proselytizing is not only to spread one's own dogmas, but inevitably also to suppress other opinions and groups.

4 Groups with pathological targets

The combination of individual pathological personality traits with negative group traits is one of the many possibilities for forming groups and developing group structures.

People with pathological personality traits can be found together in sects, racist groups ... which obviously have many, if not all of the aforementioned negative group characteristics.

In addition, there are groups that, under the guise of humanitarian aid, as representatives for others, represent their personal, conscious and unconscious interests and psychopathologies (see also: Schmidt, B. J.; Ganz, A. 2017 *„Symbiotischer Narzissmus als Gruppenphänomen"*).

Due to the motivations involved, such as attention, self-justification, pseudo-expert knowledge, information suppression and information falsification, the MSbP is maximally compatible with the corresponding negative group structures.

IV. MSBP AS A GROUP PHENOMENON

In the case of "MSbP as a group phenomenon" we are in the area of (self) help groups of parents who try to enforce the interests of their children as their representatives, real or pretended.

It should be expressly pointed out that the vast majority of parent groups use the positive opportunities, i.e. attention, influence, etc., to help their children and improve their situation. These groups are of paramount importance not only to the children concerned, but to society as a whole. In these groups one finds a "constructive (self) critical discourse", in contrast to a "narcissistic-destructive one" (Schmidt; Ganz 2017).

The latter, on the other hand, will be found in MSbP groups.

Once the "change in shape" from MSbP as an individual syndrome to a group phenomenon has succeeded by means of clinical social psychology, then it becomes immediately clear that all characteristics of groups, including negative ones, are used for implementation. So both to generate attention to satisfy narcissistic needs and to invent, induce or exaggerate illnesses in children.

The negative characteristics of groups such as dogmatization, restriction and falsification of information, proselytizing ... are used on the other hand to deceive other caregivers and the public.

On the other hand, the analysis of these groups opens up new perspectives, because as a result of the group formation, not only the individual doctor or psychologist must be deceived, but science and therapy facilities as a whole. This necessarily leads to the formation of complementary groups in these areas, i.e. in science and therapy, which at least complement the MSbP group system. But it also becomes clear that damage is no longer only done to one's own children primarily by the mothers, but also to other families and their autistic children through the MSbP groups and their complementary structures.
And it is becoming apparent that MSbP is not as rare as previously assumed.

"Although falsified medical conditions are difficult to recognize and treat, falsified conditions occurring in other settings, such as schools or mental health settings, are equally or even more complicated to address."
[Schreier et al. 2018]

1   Vulnerability ./. illness

Using an example, the difference between a vulnerability and an illness will be briefly presented.

The genetic variant of a combination of red-blonde hair and light skin is basically an adaptation to low solar radiation. This enables the body to produce appropriate vitamins even when there is little sunlight.

In an environment with high solar radiation, however, this adaptation becomes a vulnerability for the development of sunburn.

If sunburns occur more frequently in a person, this in turn increases the risk of skin cancer. Skin cancer is then a disease.

If one did not know these connections, one could well invent a disease. Since the frequency and severity of sunburns, as well as the frequency of occurrence of skin cancer, are very different, this invented disease is called "sunburn skin cancer spectrum disorder".

In the area of "autism spectrum disorder", the causal connection between autism as a vulnerability (see appendix), the resulting high probability of a "disorder of social interaction", which in turn could lead to various "profound developmental disorders", was unknown in the 1960s. These developmental disorders can in turn lead to a further disruption of social interaction, e.g. speaking is not learned. This can then lead to further disruptions in development.

Autism was particularly well suited to inventing a congenital, incurable disease.

2   Autism - the made-up disease

In the 1970s, autism was "invented" as a disease (as opposed to actual vulnerability), primarily by people who were both parents of autistic children and psychologists (Rimland, Wing). Since autism was a very rare diagnosis at the time, they only had to fool themselves - in their dual role as parents and scientists at the same time.

In the years that followed, it was often parents in this dual role who pointed the way negatively. The DAN! Project (Defeat autism now!) described in Chapter VI.2.1 is an example of this.

In several ways, autism was particularly "suitable" for MSbP.

On the one hand, the etiology of the disorders occurring, both in the area of social interaction and development, was not known at the time. The foundations for this were not yet available in the field of social psychology (Schmidt 2020).

„The carer may report a named diagnosis even when this has not been confirmed. Examples include diagnoses that are difficult to confirm or have disputed aetiology ..."
[Davis et al. 2019]

On the other hand, disorders of a psychological nature (some of which already exist) are in principle much better "suitable" for the MSbP.

"..., learning, developmental, behavioral, and psychiatric problems are even easier to exaggerate, simulate, exacerbate, coach, and induce than most physical symptoms and disability due to the heavy reliance on caregiver report for diagnosis. Caregiver reports may be the only source of information in diagnostic situations in which there are few objective diagnostic tests and the presenting problem is episodic in nature. Thus, mental health clinicians are urged not to prematurely dismiss warning signs (APSAC Taskforce, 2018)."
[Schreier et al. 2018]

And that both in the area of exaggeration and the generation of symptoms.

"There may be an insistent quest for a diagnosis. The carer may limit the child's daily activities including

school attendance. By focusing on the child's ill-health, the carer will, sometimes inadvertently, convey this to the child who may become increasingly anxious about, or come to believe in their own ill-health. This direct harm to the child is a form of emotional abuse. Indirect harm is caused by the involvement of doctors." [Davis et al. 2019]

The negative categorization of the child through the assertion that it is mentally ill, the behavior and thus also the development of the child is negatively influenced, and this is how mental disorders in the sense of a "self-fulfilling diagnosis" can be generated in the first place.

3   Origin of the dogma system

The emergence of both the "autism as an incurable disease" dogma system and the corresponding MSbP groups, as well as the interactions between the two areas, can be well classified in terms of time and geography (see also: Schmidt 2020).

GB   1962: Establishing the
        „National Autistic Society"

USA   Rimland, B. (1964): Infantile Autism

USA   1965 Autism Society of America (ASA) (former-
ly called "National Society for Autistic Children")
was founded by Bernard Rimland and Ivar Lovaas

GB   Wing, J. K. (1966): Early childhood autism. Clinical, educational and social aspects. [1st ed.].

USA   1967 Autism Research Institute (ARI) was founded by Bernard Rimland

GB   Wing, L. (1976): Early childhood autism. Clinical, educational and social aspects. [2nd ed.]

At least until 1966, the year the first edition of Wing
"Early Childhood Autism" was published, an open, helpful exchange regarding autism will be maintained, and
not only in England.
Then leads in the US
• the publication of Rimland (1964),
• the establishment of the ASA (1965) by Rimland and
Lovaas,
• as well as the ARI (1967),
• associated with the invention of the "refrigerator mother
myth" (Schmidt 2019b)
• as well as a "parent blaming" (Schmidt 2020),

to a dogmatization and at the same time the formation of MSbP groups.

Under the influence of developments in the USA, as can be proven in the second edition of Wing (1976), a dogmatic attitude towards autism is followed in England (Schmidt 2020).

The dogma system established at the time not only fulfills all the criteria of a collective MSbB, but still dominates both research / theory (Schmidt 2016, 2020) and practice / therapy (Schmidt 2017a) in the field of autism.

V. EXCURSUS: THE POWER OF THE ORGANIZATION

The importance and necessity of clinical social psychology becomes clear when the combination of pathological behavior and group structures is to be examined.

A special form of group, the organization, should be emphasized here.

If, as social psychology shows, groups are normally formed unconsciously through adaptation and imitation, this is different with organizations.

Here, a group structure is built up systematically and on a rational basis, even if it can be influenced by unconscious elements (Wetherell 1996).

If pathological, irrational behavior is institutionalized in an organization, then a pathological-irrational content is brought into a systematic, rational form.

As a result, the viewer experiences a "cognitive dissonance" (Festinger), since the pathological and irrational of the content must be brought into harmony with the rational elements of the form.

The endeavor to resolve the dissonance will in most cases lead to a failure to perceive the pathological-irrational content that would be perceived immediately outside the context of the rational organization.

For example, that children are dogmatically denied the possibility of development, although the developmental ability of people generally only ends with (brain) death. The combination of pathological-irrational behavior and rational organization necessarily goes hand in hand with a dogmatization of the content.

VI. MSBP IN AUTISM "THEORY" AND "THERAPY"

Both groups in general and the special form of organizations are dynamic structures. These arise, develop and pass away.

The characteristics of a group or organization can only be analyzed from a development perspective. This is also the case with organized forms of MSbP, for example in the area of autism.

The structure of the dogma system in the field of autism has already been presented in detail in Schmidt (2020) from the perspective of the psychology of science.

Here the dogmatization of the MSbP symptoms should be considered.

1   Denial of responsibility

It all started with the book "Infantile Autism" by Rimland (1964). The main aim of this is to exclude parents from being responsible for the behavioral and developmental disorders of autistic children.

For this purpose, Rimland on the one hand rejected the possibility of a "psychogenic" cause, both primary and

secondary. At the same time, Rimland speculated extensively about genetic and biochemical causes.

2   Chronic illness

To deny the responsibility for the education and treatment
of behavioral and developmental disorders of autistic
children, autism was dogmatized as a purely genetic or
biochemical disease that cannot be influenced by psychotherapeutic interventions.
Thus - as a consequence of the denial of responsibility - a
"chronic illness" was produced which enabled parents to
take on the role of self-sacrificing helper to an incurable
child.

*"Usually recognized as a form of child maltreatment, the
typical motivation for a parent to harm a child in this
way is to assume the "sick role" vicariously and get attention and nurturance for being a longsuffering parent
of a chronically ill child."*
[Frye; Feldman 2011]

This role, ultimately created by Rimland, was obviously
so attractive to a sufficiently large number of parents that
shortly after the publication of the book by Rimland
(1964), Lovaas and Rimland founded the ASA (1965).

3   Immunization and discrediting

It was only through the ASA that the parents and the dogma of the disease were immunized.

With the invention of the "refrigerator mother myth" (Schmidt 2019b) and the unjustified accusation of "blaming the parents" (Schmidt 2020) against science, not only the dogma was immunized against criticism. But at the same time science in general and social and developmental approaches in particular were discredited.

As a result, parents declared themselves to be the actual experts and gained the authority to interpret them.

"FII inevitably involves the carer and the child. We use 'carer' to include any primary caregiver. Most cases involve mothers. Fathers or male carers are seldom solely involved. They may collude with or be sidelined by the 'expert' mother." [Davis et al. 2019]

Until today, half a century, parents have dominated the research directions and "therapy" offers through corresponding organizations. These "therapies", as will be discussed, are highly organized forms of MSbP, child abuse, and child maltreatment.

4   Funding and ignoring

As organized groups it was possible to raise large sums of money with which
• lobbying,
• publicity campaigns,
• as well as research (e.g. through the ARI founded by Rimland in 1967)
could be carried out.
On the one hand, the need for attention was satisfied, on the other hand, it also meant that research in the autism field was and is financially well above average. As a result, there was a very large amount of research projects and publications, but
• without results because
• only in the interests of the parent organizations,
• so only in the area of genetics and biochemistry

„Bishop (2010) reported that autism prevalence and severity are comparable to those of Down syndrome, yet funding autism is six times the amount allocated to study Down syndrome. Bishop also noted, 'the slope showing increase of NIH funding over time is dramatically higher than for any other condition. It seems likely that govern-

*ment initiatives play a large role in explaining the extra-
ordinary rise of publications in autism' ."*
[Waterhouse 2013]

And Waterhouse rightly criticizes that the amount of publications does not promote knowledge about autism - on
the contrary, it hinders it. From the perspective of MSbP
as a group phenomenon, one should assume conscious
prevention.
Autism research is arguably one of the best financially
and therefore also best equipped - and at the same time
most unsuccessful.

4.1   Ignoring alternative theories and therapies

Organizations such as ASA, Autism Speaks and Autism
Germany also consistently pursued the goal that alternative approaches, both in theory and therapy, were ignored, suppressed and discredited. As shown in Schmidt
(2020), the second edition of Wing "Early childhood
autism" (1976) contains most of the alternative approaches available at the time, both in the field of therapy
and research.
But even today all "psychogenic" theories and therapies
are ignored or discredited. There is no constructive (self)
critical discourse, instead there is narcissistic-destructive

communication (see Schmidt 2016, 2017a).

Everything is possible – as long as it harms the children or at least doesn't help.

5 Separation

The "success" of the combination of pathological behavior with dogmatically secured parent organizations is the separation of autism research and therapy from psychology. Autism exists as a separate area to which the findings of developmental and social psychology, according to dogma, are not applicable, and therefore are not applied.

If one detaches the assumptions from the dogma system of the parent organizations and looks at them in the normal context of psychology, ie if one overcomes the "power of the organization" (excursus Chapter V), then the pathological properties become immediately visible.

6 Lack of valid diagnosis

After the points presented so far, it is no longer surprising that there is still no valid diagnosis (Waterhouse 2016). But it is precisely this lack of a diagnosis that opens the door, not just for pseudo-diagnoses in the form of an S3 guideline by DGKJP et al. (Vllasaliu 2016).

Parents are also given the opportunity to diagnose all possible behavioral and developmental disorders in their children with the "diagnosis" of autism.

"Symptoms reported may include challenging behaviour, autistic traits, pain, allergies, epileptic fits or gastrointestinal problems including feeding difficulties, abdominal pain and constipation. The carer may report a named diagnosis even when this has not been confirmed. Examples include diagnoses that are difficult to confirm or have disputed aetiology ..."
[Davis et al. 2019]

And at the same time the lack of a valid diagnosis serves to defend the "incurability dogma".
Because children who have largely lost their autistic symptoms (by restoring social interaction and thus development), autism was and is subsequently denied.
Autism is dogmatically considered incurable. So whoever is cured cannot be autistic.

VII. FORMS OF ILL-TREATMENT

If one assumes an existing "disorder of social interaction" and a "profound developmental disorder" as initially present, one can in principle differentiate between two forms of abuse - doing and not doing. In the area of autism, one can also differentiate between non-indicated and contra-indicated interventions.

The non-indicated ones also have massive "side effects", but the contra-indicated ones cause further symptoms or worsen existing ones.

All three forms, i.e. omission, non-indicated as well as contra-indicated interventions, are to be regarded as child abuse.

The motivation of the perpetrators, both in the case of omission as well as contra- or non-indicated therapies, is at least the fixation, if not even the deterioration of the child's condition.

"Some victims have genuine conditions and impairments that are intentionally exaggerated, undertreated, or exacerbated by the abuser. In such cases, symptoms may be exaggerated or medication may be withheld to give the impression of a treatment resistant problem."
[Schreier et al. 2018]

It will come as no surprise that all three of the aforementioned forms of abuse are not only found in autism organizations, but dominate them.

1   Omission

An essential component of failing to provide assistance to children with impaired social interaction and development is ignoring the suffering of these children. And that if left untreated, these ailments can continue into adulthood.

„*The current state of society presents an alarming prospect for those with autism:*
- low quality of life when it comes to health
- a high risk of becoming a victim of bullying, exploitation, and/or violence
- an increased risk for physical and psychological illnesses
- a significantly increased risk of dying early
- increased risk of suicide
And, particularly when it comes to sexuality and relationships:
- a high risk of becoming a victim of physical or sexual abuse" [Schmidt, et al. 2017]

47

On the basis of ignoring, the vulnerability of autistic people is glorified as a special feature, as "neurodiversity". This is propagated both by parents through books and blogs, associations of autistic people, for example "Aspies eV", as well as scientists and journalists under book titles such as "Uniquely human" (Prizant; Meyer), "Neurotribes" (Silberman), as well as various books by Theunissen on the subject of "Empowerment" ...
The result is the prevention of effective help.

"... the carer's behaviour is compounding the problems by insisting on continued investigations and a quest for a diagnosis instead of supporting a rehabilitative approach to restore the child to optimal functioning. These children's lives may be unnecessarily restricted to an extreme degree as a result of reported medical symptoms, alongside a remarkable lack of objective medical evidence of illness." [Davis et al. 2019]

The neurodiversity movement calls for autistic people to be accepted in their "uniqueness" instead of enabling them to lead a self-determined and healthy life through aids such as those offered by "child-centered programs".

2   Biochemical "interventions"

The autism dogma initiated by Rimland only excludes "psychogenic" causes and psychotherapeutic interventions, but leaves room for all other ideas of supposedly effective therapies, and even favors them.
So it is not surprising that the biochemical "treatments" - also generally found in the individual form of MSbP - occur, from diets to poisoning (e.g. using the highly corrosive substance MMS, the "Miracle Mineral Supplement").

"We present 17 children from 11 families with the allergic form of Meadow's syndrome.
In all cases their mothers believed that they had severe disease due to allergies-in 16 cases to foods and in one to house dust mite. The maternal obsession with allergen avoidance resulted in bizarre diets and life styles. Most mothers were articulate and middle class, and many had marital problems (three single parents). They had a limpet-like attachment to their child and insisted on many medical consultations. Management proved very difficult and despite careful exclusion of allergic disease, many remained on diets and failed allergy clinic follow up. In

most cases the obsession with allergy had been initiated by doctors." [Warner 1984]

All forms of abuse through biochemical treatments can still be found today in a sprawling literature on the "cure" of autism
- diets
- discharge of pollutants from the environment or vaccination
- treatment with miracle drugs like MMS
- ...

The foundations for this were laid by Rimland's book (1964) and consolidated, published and propagated by the ARI founded by Rimland (in the form of the "Defeat Autism Now!" Project).

2.1   DAN! as an example of biochemical "therapies"

The DAN! Project is a frightening example of a collective abuse of children that has been organized by parents over the years.
The number of parents involved in 2009 by ARI is frightening!

„In 2009, ARI reported that data had been collected from more than 27,000 parents ..." [Barrett 2015]

And even if Barret (2015) does not recognize the fundamental problem and is deceived about the pathological content by the rational form of organizations such as ASA and ARI, he therefore also uncritically refers to the Wikipedia entry regarding Rimland's "merits" in the fight against the "Parent blaming", and describes ABA as a scientifically proven treatment, his presentation of the DAN! project is so detailed that the central points are cited here:

"The DAN! project, which was launched in 2005, grew out of discussions between Rimland, Jon Pangborn, Ph.D., and Sidney MacDonald Baker, M.D., all of whom had become interested in nonstandard approaches to treating autistic children. Rimland and Pangborn both had family members who were autistic." [Barrett 2015]

"The "DAN! protocol" was centered around the belief that autism is caused by a combination of lowered immune response; external toxins from vaccines and other sources; and problems caused by certain foods. The underlying philosophy, which was posted to the Center for

*the Study of Autism Web Web site for several years, inclu-
ded the following ideas:*
*Autism and related problems are the symptoms of dys-
function of the neural, immune and/or digestive systems
which occur in individuals genetically sensitive to such
factors as sub-optimal nutrition, food intolerances, mi-
crobial overgrowth and toxins. Appropriate treatment
entails identifying and alleviating the problems causing
the symptoms in that individual, rather than merely att-
empting to suppress the symptoms through the use of psy-
choactive drugs."* [Barrett 2015]

*"In 1995, ARI sponsored a 3-day meeting that was atten-
ded by about 30 professionals who discussed what they
were doing and what they believed had worked for them.
These determinations were not derived from well-desig-
ned studies but were based on clinical impressions, observations reported by parents to the treating physicians,
and responses to questionnaires that ARI had collected.
The meeting generated a consensus document—co-aut-
hored by Baker and Pangborn—that was published in
1996 as Biomedical Assessment Options for Children
with Autism and Related Problems, but was often referred to as the DAN! Clinical Manual" or DAN! Protocol." In 2005, after undergoing five revisions, the report
was extensively rewritten, revised once more, and publis-*

hed by ARI as a large book called Autism: Effective Bio-medical Treatments. The original version of the book co-vered 41 pages. The 2005 version, ..., has about 330 pa-ges ..." [Barrett 2015]

"DAN!'s Mercury Detoxification Position Paper
DAN!'s most harmful activities were its promotion of che-lation therapy and opposition to vaccination. In 2001, DAN! convened a Detoxification Consensus Conference and issued a position paper which claimed that mercury in some vaccines could cause autism and that treating autistic children with chelation therapy could cause many of them to improve. The paper was supported in part by a grant from Kirkman Laboratories. Following another conference, the paper was updated in 2005. Both versions of the statement claim (falsely) that "body bur-den" of mercury can be measuring the urinary mercury concentration after a chelating drug is administered. This procedure, called provoked or challenge testing, has been denounced as meaningless by the American College of Medical Toxicologists and labeled as "below the stan-dard of care" by the Oregon Medical Board. The 2005 version of the DAN! mercury-detoxification paper also stated that children can be exposed to mercury through maternal seafood consumption, maternal dental fillings (amalgam), and childhood vaccines." [Barrett 2015]

In the DAN! Project, it is again parents who, as supposed experts, initiate and justify the abuse of children.

"Rimland, Baker, and many others have asserted that ARI's parental reports are evidence that the treatments are effective. But that is absolutely untrue."
[Barrett 2015]

But all of these ideas regarding what causes and cures autism still exist unchallenged. And autistic children are still mistreated under the pretext of "healing" with sense-less diets and dangerous biochemical attempts at healing. However, doing the wrong thing usually also means failing to do what is helpful.

3   "Behavioral Therapies"

Due to the denial of the parents' responsibility for the be-havioral and developmental disorders of their children, and the resulting rejection of any psychogenic causation, all existing and future psychosocial and psychotherapeu-tic treatment and support approaches had to be discred-ited and excluded .
In order to fill this vacuum, treatments were required that were completely free of any psychosocial components.

On the one hand, the ABA developed by Lovaas, the "Applied Behavior Analysis", and on the other hand the "TEACCH" developed by Schopler were available.

3.1   ABA

Bernard Rimland founded the ASA in 1965 together with Ivar Lovaas, the inventor of this treatment, which had no psychotherapeutic content and which in principle could not lead to an improvement in the children. The supposed therapy, which is only a pseudo-scientific form of abuse, was implemented in the parents' organization right from the start. And is still dominant, even if it is used today under many other names. For decades, and wrongly, ABA was considered the "gold standard" (e.g. autismus Deutschland e.V. 2016), while today in Germany the newer, better-sounding forms such as the "Early Start Denver Model" are preferred.

Detached from the context of the seriousness and rationality mediating organizations and the dogma systems anchored there, the irrationality becomes immediately clear.

Outside of autism, no developmental and social psychologist or linguist would come up with the idea or confirm that one could treat disorders of social communication and development through ABA. With ABA as a maximally intensive treatment which, carried out over several hours a day, prevents the development in natural social coexistence and thereby creates, intensifies or fixes the symptoms in the first place.

As early as 1967 Bruno Bettelheim wrote in his book *"The Empty Fortress"*:

„Here I wish also to comment on current efforts to deal with infantile autism through operant conditioning—that is, by creating conditioned responses through punishment and reward. Temporarily this breaks down the child's defenses against experiencing the frustrations of reality and arouses him to some action. But the actions are not of his devising. They are those the experimenter wants; that is, they are conditioned response actions. Which means that autistic children are reduced to the level of Pavlovian dogs. ...

According to a recent description of operant conditioning [Lovaas, Berberich, PerioflF, SchaeflFer, 1966]:
Training was conducted six days a week, seven hours a day, with a fifteen-minute rest period accompanying each hour of training. During the training sessions the child and the adult sat facing each other, their heads about thirty cm apart. The adult physically prevented the child from leaving the training situation by holding the child's legs between his own legs. Rewards, in the form of single

spoonsful of the child's meal, were delivered immediately after correct responses. Punishment (spanking, shouting by the adult) was delivered for inattentive, self-destructve, and tantrumous behavior which interfered with the training, and most of these behaviors were thereby supressed within one week. ...

Speech in the sense of communication simply cannot be forced out of children. It can only be acquired as the outcome of personal relations. Forcing them into echolalia by bribing, shouting, or spanking will only lead to a greater dehumanization.

[Bettelheim 1967]

It was probably also this criticism of ABA that led to Bettelheim being subsequently discredited by Rimland and his supporters using the "refrigerator mother myth" (Schmidt 2019b).

Social interaction is learned through social interaction. Language develops in a complex interaction from the maturation of the child in and with his environment (see e.g. Vygotsky 1981, 1983, 1987, 1993).

A daily training of the child for several hours is abuse - no matter what name it takes.

The parent organizations have not only propagated this form of abuse and are still propagating it, they are displacing other, helpful therapeutic approaches through ignorance and discrediting.

"Nevertheless, the long-term negative impact of thwarted developmental milestones, developmentally inappropriate socialization, incorrect self-perceptions of ability and functioning, or iatrogenic harm from medications designed to treat behavioral disorders can be profound."
[Schreier et al. 2018]

What is offered or recommended as treatments by the parent organizations creates or solidifies the problems as a form of organized MSbP.

"Available data suggests that caregiver with MSBP is usually victim's mother.
Most commonly these women have others mental disorders. MSBP is a very dangerous form of violence and it is proven that the mortality associated with this disorder reaches about 6-33%. It should be noted that, in addition to the obvious child's physical injuries, abnormal relationships with caregiver cause long-term developmental damages." [Zarankiewicz et al. 2019]

The results of a large study from Sweden are reproduced without comment:

*„In this large population-based study, we observed incre-
ased mortality in individuals with ASD. Mortality was increased in both low-functioning and high-functioning
ASD, as well as in both genders. ...
The observed OR [odds ratio] of 2.56 for ASD in relation
to all-cause mortality is in line with most of the previous
clinical and population-based mortality studies. We
found that increased mortality in ASD was not limited to
certain causes of death, such as diseases of nervous system, but was elevated for all analysed categories according to the ICD, apart from infectious diseases."*
[Hirvikoski et al. 2016]

3.2   TEACCH

The idea that a well-structured environment is helpful for
teaching children with learning disabilities is by no
means new, but was developed further by Eric Schopler
into TEACCH (Treatment and Education of Autistic and
related Communication handicapped Children).
Schopler and TEACCH were part of the "English direc-
tion" around Lorna Wing and her husband John.
As *a* means, as a ***means***, TEACCH makes sense. But in
the context of the autism dogma of the non-treatable and
also non-educable autistic child, the goal was taken from
the means and became THE means.

Comparable to a surgeon who casts all of his patients' injured limbs in plaster, regardless of the type and severity of the injuries.

VIII. THE MSBP SYSTEM

With MSbP as a group phenomenon, the motives, actions and concomitants present in the individual form are distributed among several actors in a system. These actors in turn sometimes form sub-groups, which can simulate the independence of different perspectives.

The dissociation within a perpetrator described by Feldmann (1994) is thus shifted to the entire group, the MSbP system.

The different motives - such as satisfying the needs for recognition and attention, for effectiveness, suppression of reality and denial of responsibility, career and profit - appear distributed among the actors and subgroups and in different combinations.

Actions such as inventing or exaggerating a diagnosis, carrying out abuse, deception ... are also taken over by the various actors and subgroups.

Concomitant phenomena such as proselytizing, suppression and falsification of information, ... are also divided up, making them more difficult to perceive and analyze.

The MSbP system offers the same advantage over scientific perception and analysis as a flock of birds or fish over the predator.

In the following, the structures and relationships are

shown using the parent organization "Autismus Deutsch-land e.V.", which has existed for 50 years, as an example, so to speak as a case description.

There are three groups that are closely related to autism Germany:

- parents
- Doctors, psychologists, researchers ...
- Autistic self-advocates

These three groups are closely and reciprocally connected through assessors.

Doubt about the supposed autonomy is more than justi-fied.

IX. PARENTS AS ORGANIZED GROUPS

Not all parents of autistic children are organized in a group. And not all parents who are in a corresponding organization, be it self-help group, parent forum ..., have the MSbP.

Originally, however, the autism organizations that are dominant today emerged from parents who primarily refused to share responsibility for their children's development / behavior problems (Schmidt 2020).

And parents with MSbP will find ideal conditions in appropriate groups.

"The perpetrator may seek emotional and sometimes material support from wider family members and, increasingly, through social media." [Davis et al. 2019]

and

"People, who suffer from this disease take part in support groups. During the meetings they not only take the identity of a child's caregiver, but also receive the compassion and attention of the group's participants. This is a psycho reward for them (Janus, 2015). In most of the cases, the

perpetrator is a parent (most often a mother) and the victim is a child." [Majda et al. 2019]

as well Frye and Feldman:

"These parents can receive attention by attending numerous support groups for parents with disabled children as an experienced veteran who has dealt with the disability in their child and overcome it (Ayoub et al. 2002)."
[Frye; Feldman 2011]

The children of parents with MSbP can be divided into two groups. On the one hand in autistic children, who therefore have a corresponding vulnerability (see appendix) and, because of this vulnerability, have their first communication and development disorders.
On the other hand there are children who do not have autism.
The parents of these children created the diagnosis of autism in the first place, whether in the presence or absence of behavioral problems in the child, in order to satisfy their own needs.

"Ayoub et al. (2002b) presented the case studies of two parents who requested that their children be referred for special education, even though the children's teachers

found no basis for concern. One mother referred her two younger daughters after her oldest son was placed in special education due to behaviors related to Asperger's syndrome. With both younger children, the mother insisted on evaluations by school professionals and independent evaluations paid for by the school district. Medical testing by physicians accompanied the educational assessments. All results indicated no physical ailments or learning problems. In spite of these results, the middle child was taking Ritalin for ADHD and the youngest child was placed in the same special education school her brother attended." [Frye; Feldman 2011]

and

"*Ayoub et al. (2002) also briefly described nine children from five families who were identified as displaying "educational condition falsification" (ECF). Eight of the nine children were diagnosed with ADHD. Children in this sample were also falsely identified as having learning disabilities (usually language-based disorders), psychiatric illnesses, and behavioral disorders. In three of the five families, more than one child was a victim of ECF or PCF. The mothers in each of the families were depicted as demanding and adversarial in their dealings with school personnel.*

The parents in these cases were depicted by Ayoub et al. (2002) as 'bold, insistent, and at times quite adversarial in their demands of the school.

...

She identified herself as the parent of a child with autism and spoke for an extended length of time, explaining her child's needs.

The special education director from the local school district recognized her and privately followed up on the parent's report to ensure that the student was getting proper services.

The director learned that the student was receiving special education, but was not identified as a student with autism. The director requested some informal observations of the student by a school psychologist and a clinical psychologist to confirm that there were no indications of autism. One of the student's teachers reported that the student's family was well able to take care of the child without public aid (name withheld by request, July 2011, personal communication)." [Frye; Feldman 2011]

1   Parents' motivations

It cannot be stressed enough that there is of course no one-to-one relationship between membership in a support group and MSbP. Not all parents in self-help groups have

MSbP, and autistic vulnerability is often, if not always, real. Parents have a wide variety of motivations to get involved in a self-help group.

1.1   Healthy motivation - help for the child

The normal and healthy attitude of parents is the desire to help their own child optimally and to put their own needs behind those of the child. This healthy motivation and attitude can also be found both inside and outside of self-help groups. It can even be assumed that this is the most common motivation of all.

1.2   Morbid motivations

The pathological motivations are those described in the MSbP:

"*We can determine three types of mothers.*
First type, a mother who looks for a help. She expects interest and attention from a medical personnel. She comes from pathological family and has experienced a violence. Her pregnancy was unexpected and often raises a child on her own. She mainly agrees with a diagnosis, child's treatment and for a foster family.

Second type, a mother an 'active perpetrator'. She is able to use a very aggressive and harmful methods toward a child. She is characterized by being emotionally unstable, depression and strong denial mechanism.
Third type, a mother who feels a need to be the most important person during a treatment. She has a medical knowledge, suggests her own solutions to doctors, tries to mislead them, so as a consequence she can undermining doctors competences. She feels important and that is her goal to gain." [Majda et al. 2019]

These pathological motivations can also be found in corresponding parent groups, organizations and MSbP systems. Due to the motivations regarding attention, effectiveness, repression, etc., which go far beyond the healthy desire for help for their own child, parents with MSbP dominate most self-help groups.

2 Autismus Deutschland e.V. as an an example

> *You should recognize them by their deeds!*
> *(1. Johannes 2,1-6)*

"Autismus Deutschland e.V" was founded around 50 years ago and today controls the autism area in Germany.

This through financing and / or influencing both direct and indirect, on regional parent groups, own and external therapy centers, as well as "research".

The typical characteristics of MSbP can also be found here.

2.1   Striving for attention

The immense financial resources over the decades have been and are being invested in "Autism Awareness", in activities that generate attention and thus generate donations again.

No other physical or mental disability / vulnerability is as present in the public as the "Autism Spectrum Disorder".

2.2   Pretend Help

However, it does not provide effective aid aimed at improving disorders of social communication and development. Instead, with a great deal of resources, help is only faked, as already explained in detail in Schmidt (2017a).

"A mother, who suffers from the MSbP is very loving and caring. She does not leave her child during the hospitalization. She also makes relationship with a medical per-

sonnel; she treats them like friends, they admire her for her devotion and medical knowledge. Recognition and admiration is what she was expected to get, she feels satisfied. Nevertheless, in the reality a child is being rejected by a mother." [Majda et al. 2019]

What Majda et al describes for mothers is adopted by Autismus Deutschland. Fake help as a means of gaining attention and recognition.

2.3 Preventing effective aid

Due to the dominance of Autismus Deutschland e.V. at all levels, parent organizations, therapy centers, etc., parents of autistic children automatically and without alternative come into contact with the MSbP structures of Autismus Deutschland e.V. Even the many families who are seriously looking for help for their autistic children only receive offers of useless or harmful "information" and "therapies".

2.4 Suppression and discrediting of helpful information

Anything that could help autistic children and their parents is suppressed or discredited.

This happens through one-sided information, which is so massively scattered and repeated by the substructures that other positions are hardly visible.

The dogma of the incurably ill child with self-sacrificing parents is reflected in many ways, like the echo in a cave, through books, regional groups, forums, internet groups, etc. This information is given the appearance of seriousness by doctors and psychologists as accomplices.

X. DOCTORS / PSYCHOLOGISTS AS (CO-) PERPETRATORS

At the beginning, parents and researchers were in personal union - these roles were also dissociated in the following years. In parents on the one hand, and doctors and psychologists on the other. Participation in the MSbP system, as well as the importance for the delimitation, stability and expansion of the same, can be seen in three points:

1. psychological primitivism
2. the lack of professional distance
3. the active invention and induction of diseases

At the same time, it becomes clear that not only the primary caregivers can be the perpetrators of child abuse within an MSbP system, but also people who have a guarantor position due to their education, social position (e.g. as professors) and state funding.

1   Psychological primitivism

The conformity demanded of their members by groups is "normal" even among psychologists etc. (West 1981). But the "psychological primitivism" that has existed for

50 years indicates a pronounced psychopathy of the researchers involved.

The control compulsion inherent in behaviorism as a
whole is transferred to autism "theories" and "therapies".

1.1   Behaviorism

Even if operant conditioning, e.g. increased reactions to a
stimulus through rewards, occurs in learning, behaviorism has been criticized as an ideology with the claim to
sole representation since the 1960s and is no longer taken
seriously in psychological circles today.

Anyone who, as a psychologist, still adheres to behavior-
istic thinking, and thus ABA in all its manifestations as
"therapy", has suppressed or ignored the development of
psychology over the last 50 years.

Yet the area of autism is still dominated by behaviorism
in both theory and practice.

1.2   Static instead of dynamic development

In order to exclude both primary and secondary responsibility for communication and developmental disorders in
children and at the same time to satisfy the need for a
chronically ill child, in the early 1970s autistic children
were dogmatically denied any development opportunities

(Schmidt 2020). On the basis of these dogmas, the "profound developmental disorder" is still considered static, that is, as a postulate instead of a problem (Schmidt 2020). The application of any knowledge of developmental psychology was also categorically excluded.

1.3   Isolated instead of social psychological

The "disturbance of social interaction" was and is, also following the dogma, considered to be caused in isolation in the child. The fact that even children born deaf-blind are willing and able to interact socially was ignored. The results of social psychology, especially with regard to unconscious group communication using facial expressions, gestures, language (dialects, modulation, ...), but also language development, concept development ... have not been and are not used.

1.4   Hindsight-bias on diagnosis

In addition to the many other methodological errors in autism research, which were already presented in Schmidt 2015a and 2015b, the hindsight error should be briefly discussed here, as this in turn is the basis for the invention and induction of illness.
From the finding that diagnosed autistic children already

showed behavioral problems in early childhood (retro-spect), it is derived, conversely, that all children with be-havioral problems in early childhood are also autistic and will develop disorders of communication and develop-ment (error!). The mistreatment of children is justified by means of the hindsight mistake, which should not occur in the case of doctorates in medicine and psychology, as will be presented in the section on "induced illness".

2   Lack of professional distance

The lack of professional distance is both necessary and characteristic of the involvement of doctors and psychol-ogists as perpetrators in the MSbP system.

"While some of the carer's behaviour causes direct harm to the child by emotional and/or physical abuse or ne-glect, the involvement of doctors is central within FII. The doctor(s) often, although inadvertently, cause or al-low much of the harm suffered by the child. Reliance on carer reports of history and diagnoses, and accepting the carer as a conduit of medical information is based on pa-ediatricians' default assumptions regarding parents' trut-hfulness and reliability—'mother knows best', described by Kahneman as System 1 thinking." [Davis et al. 2019]

This is shown by the "scientific advisory board" at Autismus Deutschland, which is largely congruent with "WGAS-Autismus".
But there are also associations between individual scientists and parent groups.

"Most importantly, experience suggests that much of FII becomes a major problem when doctors accept the carer's 'offer' of illness , even though their clinical judgement suggests otherwise. In doing so they can inadvertently collude with the carer in a way that has damaging consequences for the child, whose needs become subsumed by the needs of the carer." [Davis et al. 2019]

The alliance between "scientists" and parents in the area of MSbP necessarily leads to the fact that the needs of the children are no longer perceived and that action is taken against them.
Scientists, for whom the well-being of the children was the top priority, were accused of "blaming the parents" (Schmidt 2020), as the Tinbergens had to learn.

"Before we consider the possibility [of psychogenic factors] in more detail, we must remember that many people have non-scientific, non-rational reasons for rejecting the psychogenic hypothesis. As we shall discuss in a

moment, part (though by no means all) of the psycho-genic factors are to do with the behaviour of the parents, in particular the mother. It is of course extremely painful to have to believe that one may have contributed to the catastrophe that has hit one's child; even if there is no question of blame, the awareness or even a suspicion of such a possibility inevitably gives rise to feelings of guilt. These make it emotionally almost impossible for parents of autistic children to accept the theory of a psychogenic origin of autism, even in the face of quite suggestive evi-dence. Not only is there such non-rational resistance against this idea particularly, and a wish for either a genetic or another accident to be at the root of autism, but parents, again quite naturally, feel that adherents of the psychogenic thesis are cruel to them. As Dr L. Wing has told us several times: 'you are hard on mothers'. When we nevertheless publish what we consider to be a good case for a mainly environmental, and mainly psy-chogenic, origin of autism, we do this because the child-ren's chances of recovery – or of being protected from even becoming autistic – are enhanced by therapies deri-ved from this insight; and the children's interest must come first. If we have to choose between hurting some mothers and refusing to rescue many children from the disastrous downward spiral we feel we have no choice but 'to be hard on mothers'." [Tinbergen 1983]

The doctors and psychologists who - mostly in personal union - are on the advisory board of Autismus Deutschland and WGAS-Autismus, have decided differently.

3   Induced disease

Doctors and psychologists become perpetrators by demanding and promoting the mistreatment of children on the basis of invented diagnoses, e.g. by means of "early intervention".

The position paper "On the necessity of an autism-specific early therapy" (Autismus Deutschland e.V. 2020) can be found on the website of Autismus Deutschland, which, on the basis of an invalid diagnosis, propagates the induction of developmental and communication disorders by means of contraindicated "therapies". The "scientific advisory board" is responsible for this, at least to a large extent.

„Wissenschaftliche Sicht auf Autismus-Spektrum-Störungen, frühe Diagnostik und frühe Therapie.
Autismus-Spektrum-Störungen gehören zu den tiefgreifenden Entwicklungsstörungen (ICD 10: F 84.0) und sind gekennzeichnet durch massive Beeinträchtigungen aller Entwicklungsbereiche: Störungen der Sprachentwicklung, der Kommunikation und Interaktion sowie gravie-

rende Verhaltensprobleme. Nicht bzw. falsch oder zu spät behandelt führen sie häufig zu schwerwiegenden Verhaltensstörungen, wie z.B. selbst- oder fremdverletzendem Verhalten. Je später das Kind und Eltern einen Zugang zur Autismustherapie erhalten, desto höher ist ebenfalls das Risiko der Ausbildung von Sekundärstörungen beim Kind (z.B. herausforderndes Verhalten, Schwierigkeiten bei der Beschulung) und der Erhöhung der Belastungsfaktoren bei den Eltern. Diese sind laut einiger Studien besonders stark belastet (z. B. Hoffman et al., 2009), häufig auch stärker als Eltern von Kindern mit anderen Behinderungen."[1] [autismus Deutschland e.V. 2020]

---

1   Scientific view on autism spectrum disorders, early diagnosis and early therapy.
    Autism spectrum disorders belong to the profound developmental disorders (ICD 10: F 84.0) and are characterized by massive impairments in all areas of development: disorders of language development, communication and interaction as well as serious behavioral problems. Not treated or treated incorrectly or too late often lead to serious behavioral disorders, such as self-injurious or injurious behavior. The later the child and parents have access to autism therapy, the higher the risk of developing secondary disorders in the child (e.g. challenging behavior, difficulties in schooling) and the increase in stress factors in the parents. According to some studies, these are particularly exposed to stress (e.g. Hoffman et al., 2009), often more so than parents of children with other disabilities.

There is no risk assessment. It is not investigated which damage, e.g. interaction and developmental disorders, arise or can be fixed as such by the treatments recommended below. It does not ask the simple question of what effects these "treatments" would have on undiagnosed children.

The focus is on avoiding "secondary disorders" that are stressful for the parents ...

The fact that these secondary disturbances also have other causes and can only be generated by the MSbP, for example, is not taken into account.

"Ayoub et al. (2002b) express concern that students with falsified educational difficulties are at risk for school failure and emotional problems. They noted that the students in their sample exhibited temper tantrums, out-of-control behavior, aggressive acting out, symptoms of depression, and symptoms of oppositional defiant disorder. Wilde (2004) notes that children of parents with FDP face the risk of not developing personal responsibility because of their parent's desire to keep them dependent. These children also tend to rely on their parents to shelter them from responsibility. According to a Harvard research study in progress, the longterm psychological and educational morbidities of forged educational pre-

sentations of FDP are substantial (C. Ayoub, July 2011, personal communication)." [Frye; Feldman 2011]

The occurrence of secondary disorders justifies the cause of these secondary disorders by means of MSbP, by child abuse.

3.1   No valid diagnosis

In principle, there is no valid diagnosis of autism (Waterhouse et al. 2016). And there can be no such thing when considering autism as a vulnerability.
In addition, there is the fact that all children go through phases of autistic behavior during their development, and these behaviors can also be caused by other handicaps. Often there is only a difference of degree between autistic and "normal" behavior.

"Any of the items of behaviour described above may be seen in normal children and in children with other kinds of handicaps, at some stage in their development. They can at times be withdrawn, obsessional, have temper tantrums or cling to special objects. The autistic child, however, shows the behaviour for years on end, and does virtually nothing else at all (until he begins to emerge from the illness). His oddness stands out all day and eve-

ry day, not just now and again, or when he not feeling well." [Wing, John K. 1966]

According to John K. Wing, a reliable diagnosis in early childhood is simply not possible.

"Differentiation from Normality
Most of the symptoms of childhood autism can be seen in normal children at some stage in their development. Thus, there is a time when normal children can only recognize their parents if they are fairly close and all children show echolalia during the early early stages of speech development. Hutt et al. (1965) found it difficult to distinguish between the motor behaviour of 4-year-old normal and autistic children in an unstructured environment. A few mildly autistic children may in fact develop normally in late childhood, and in their early years the syndrome may be difficult to detect. However, the behaviour shown by most young autistic children is severely abnormal because it is made up of elements which are normal only if they are transitory, and which persist all day and every day for years. It is therefore most unlikely to be missed." [Wing, John K. 1966]

Elisabeth and Niko Tinbergen also represent the perspective of a gradual difference between autistic and "normal" behavior.

"But when, in 1970, we read the statement by Drs. John and Corinne Hutt that '... apart from gaze aversion of the face, all other components of the social encounters of these autistic children are those shown by normal non-autistic children'. (13, p. 147), we suddenly sat up, because we knew from many years of child watching that normal children quite often show all the elements of Kanner's syndrome." [Tinbergen 1974]

In addition, every child is different, develops differently, develops different disorders ... and that depends on the interaction with the social environment.

"Each child has his own pattern of affected and unaffected functions. The second component in severity is due to the interaction between the primary disabilities and the environment. Even normal children brought up in some environments will be disturbed in behaviour or educationally backward (Rutter, 1972a). Handicapped children are particularly vulnerable to such harmful social milieux and need, in addition, very skilled management if an otherwise normal environment is to be of maximum va-

lue. Thus social withdrawal, disturbance in behaviour and educational backwardness may vary markedly depending both on the severity of the impairments and on the suitability of the environment." [Wing 1976]

In addition, all children have periods of defiance, show challenging behavior, go through "crises" (see Vygotsky 1998, among others).

„Die 2016 neu formulierten S3-Leitlinien (AWMF online 2016) zur Diagnostik autistischer Störungen (Handlungsempfehlungen für Mediziner und Psychologen) empfehlen für die Diagnostik von Autismus-Spektrum-Störungen das Diagnosealter von 1 ½ Jahren. Sehr genau werden in den Leitlinien die Frühsymptome geschildert, mit der Zielsetzung, früh eine gezielte Therapie initiieren zu können. Viele Eltern sind inzwischen gut informiert und kümmern sich früh um eine Diagnose ihres Kindes, um dementsprechend frühzeitig eine passgenaue Hilfe zu erhalten.“[2] [autismus Deutschland e.V. 2020]

---

2   The S3 guidelines, newly formulated in 2016 (AWMF online 2016) for the diagnosis of autistic disorders (recommendations for action for doctors and psychologists) recommend a diagnosis of 1½ years for diagnosing autism spectrum disorders. The early symptoms are described very precisely in the guidelines, with the aim of being able to initiate targeted therapy at an early stage. Many parents are now well informed and take care of a diagnosis

84

On the one hand, this statement is untenable, and it shifts the "diagnosis" to the parents' side, who are presented as "meanwhile well informed". This can be described as a direct invitation to MSbP and as a result enables "treatments" just because the parents "want" it.

The recommendation for early intervention is based, in summary, on an invalid diagnosis using "S3 guidelines" (Vllasaliu 2016), the authors of which are almost identical to the scientific advisory board of Autismus Deutschland, and are therefore responsible for the position paper as "scientists".

By means of hindsight errors and a lack of impact assessment, the same people not only define the wrong, invalid diagnostic criteria, but also recommend harmful therapies.

3.2   Disease-inducing "therapies"

On the basis of psychological primitivism and an invented diagnosis, the position paper "On the necessity of an autism-specific early therapy" recommends an intervention pot pourrie in a completely undifferentiated and uncritical manner. In the majority of cases, it can be as-

---

of their child at an early stage in order to receive tailored help at an early stage.

sumed that the child and its development are directly at risk.

„In diesem Rahmen kommen verschiedene autismusspezifische Methoden der Frühintervention bei dem Kind zum Einsatz, wie beispielsweise
- Early Start Denver Modell (ESDM)
- Frankfurter Frühinterventionsprogramm (A-FIPP)
- Aufmerksamkeits-Interaktionstherapie (AIT)
- Unterstützte Kommunikation (UK)
- Picture Exchange System (PECS)
- Structured Teaching (TEACCH)
- Floortime (DIR)
- Relationship Development Intervention (RDI)
- Differentielle Beziehungstherapie (DBT)
u.a.m."[3] [autismus Deutschland e.V. 2020]

---

3   "In this context, various autism-specific methods of early intervention are used in the child, such as
   - Early Start Denver Model (ESDM)
   - Frankfurt Early Intervention Program (A-FIPP)
   - Attention Interaction Therapy (AIT)
   - Assisted communication (UK)
   - Picture Exchange System (PECS)
   - Structured Teaching (TEACCH)
   - Floortime (DIR)
   - Relationship Development Intervention (RDI)
   - Differential Relationship Therapy (DBT)
   and others more"

3.2.a   ABA and derivatives

Some of the recommended treatments are based on ABA, even when repackaged and relabeled, such as the Early Start Denver Model.

Here children are taken out of their normal learning environment in order to be trained for hours using operant conditioning.

Anyone who, in the end necessarily, would like to consider the biological basis for the development of the child should look to the biologists or ethologists, and not the behaviorists.

"*Aus diesen Zusammenhängen können Eltern lernen: Auch wenn sie ihr Kind gezeugt haben und es darum nur von ihnen stammende Erbanlagen besitzt, so ist doch die Kombination des Erbguts neu und ganz anders als bei ihnen selbst. Daraus kann eine Persönlichkeit von völlig anderem Wesen hervorgehen, von jedem Elternteil grundverschieden. Daraus folgt: Ihr Kind, obgleich ihr eigen Fleisch und Blut, ist für Eltern ein unvorauszusehendes, unbekanntes Wesen; sie müssen alle Aufmerksamkeit daransetzen, es kennenzulernen und als eigenständige Persönlichkeit zu begreifen. Erst dann werden sie ihm gerecht werden können. ...*

Es gibt kaum ein Kind, das uns nicht dann und wann durch neue Wortschöpfungen überrascht. Durch schöpferisches Erfinden erweitern die Kinder aus eigenem Antrieb ihren Erfahrungsbereich in vielen Dimensionen. Das Kleinkind hat seine besten Lehrer in sich selbst: Es wäre hoffnungslos, seine angeborenen Lernstrategien und die dazugehörigen Motivationen durch von außen aufgeprägte Lehrpläne ersetzen zu wollen: solche können im Kleinkindalter nur stören, indem sie die zur Natur des Kindes gehörigen, viel sinnvolleren Lernstrategien verdrängen. Hier liegen die entscheidenden wissenschaftlichen Argumente gegen die von der amerikanischen Lerntheorie provozierte Forderung, lernzielorientiertes Lehren und Lernen schon in die Welt des kleinen Kindes einzuführen. ...

Unterdrückbarkeit durch Angst. Der gesamte zur Lebenstüchtigkeit und Selbständigkeit beitragende Verhaltenskomplex Erkunden/ Spielen/Nachahmen/schöpferisches Erfinden hat nun noch eine behutsame biologisch begründete Eigenschaft: Er entfaltet sich nur im Zustand der inneren Gelöstheit. Für das Spielen wird dies in der Psychologie so formuliert: »Spielen erfolgt nur im entspannten Feld.«[4] [Hassenstein 1987]

---

4   Parents can learn from these contexts: Even if they have conceived their child and therefore only has genes derived from them, the combination of the genetic material is new and completely different from their own. This can result in a personality

3.2.b   PECS

The recommendation of PECS, the "Picture Exchange and Communication System", which enables communication by exchanging picture cards, follows psychological primitivism, which turns the problems in the area of language development in autistic children into a dogmatic postulate (Schmidt 2020).

---

of a completely different nature, fundamentally different from each parent. It follows from this: Your child, although her own flesh and blood, is an unforeseeable, unknown being to parents; they must pay all their attention to get to know it and understand it as an independent personality. Only then will they be able to do justice to him. ...

There is hardly a child who does not surprise us every now and then with new word creations. Through creative invention, the children expand their area of experience in many dimensions on their own initiative. The toddler has its best teachers in itself: It would be hopeless to want to replace its innate learning strategies and the associated motivations with externally imprinted curricula: these can only be disruptive in early childhood by suppressing the much more meaningful learning strategies that are inherent in the child's nature . This is where the decisive scientific arguments lie against the demand provoked by American learning theory to introduce learning-goal-oriented teaching and learning into the world of small children. ...

Oppressibility through fear. The entire behavioral complex of exploring / playing / imitating / creative invention that contributes to fitness for life and independence now has one more cautious, biologically based property: it only develops in a state of inner relaxation. For play, this is formulated in psychology as follows: "Play only takes place in a relaxed field."

It is not asked how the problems in language development come about and how they can be eliminated, but simply replace linguistic communication with picture boards.

In this way, language development is not promoted, but rather prevented.

3.2.c   Floortime (DIR)

Amazingly, the DIR / Floortime approach is also found among the recommended interventions.

This approach is based on the restoration of social interaction by playing together with the child in a specially created "relaxed field" (see Hassenstein 1987), i.a. with the least possible stimulus, the limitation to two players, etc.

The DIR / Floortime approach was first presented in detail in German-speaking countries in Ganz, Schmidt (2016). At a time when Autismus Deutschland e.V., and against criticism from parents and autistic circles, still represented ABA as the "gold standard" (Autismus Deutschland e.V. 2016).

The actually positive mention of a constructive approach must ultimately be seen as a concealment tactic of the MSbP system. Because this approach does not fit together with ESDM and comparable ABA-based approaches.

4   Effects

Doctors and psychologists involved in the MSbP system open the door to the MSbP by means of psychological primitivism, invented diagnoses and recommendations for harmful treatments.
At the same time, they legitimize child abuse so that parents no longer have to deceive medical-psychological staff.
The "scientists" also prevent effective help because they only spread misinformation about autism and prevent scientific discourse.
However, through pseudoscientific dogmatic positions, they not only have a damaging effect on the children of MSbP parents, but also on all autistic children and their families.
The definition of "proxy" must therefore be clearly broader in the area of "MSbP as a group phenomenon".

XI. AUTISTIC SELF-ADVOCATES

In addition to the groups of parents and "scientists", there are still autistic self-advocates, either as lone fighters or organized in groups, such as ASAN (Autistic Self Advocacy Network) with the slogan "Nothing About Us Without Us", or Aspies eV in Germany . Members of Aspies e.V. can be found as assessors at both Autismus Deutschland e.V. and WGAS-Autismus, and are thus integrated into the MSbP system.

1 Motivations

The main motives of the self-advocate are the preservation and expansion of the primary and secondary gain from illness and the satisfaction of narcissistic needs. In contrast, goals regarding improvement, especially for autistic people with severe impairments, are not found, at least on a practical level.

2 Have a stabilizing effect

The self-advocacy organizations stabilize the MSbP system as they are supposedly involved in decisions and developments on behalf of other autistic people. But in the

end they only represent their own interests.
So they offer a participation alibi.

3   Prevent "abuse through treatment"

By vehemently campaigning against ABA, the self-advocates ended this form of treatment at Autismus Deutschland e.V. and stopped the financial support from Aktion
Mensch. However, this commitment was very limited in
time. There are hardly any protests against current, con-
verted forms of ABA.

4   Promote "abuse through omission"

At the same time, the self-advocacy organizations en-
courage mistreatment through omission by ignoring the
massive dangers to the physical and mental health of
autistic people on the one hand, and at the same time glo-
rifying the existing vulnerability through the neuro-diver-
sity dogma.
Autism is also presented as untreatable by these organizations. This encourages abuse through omission - in line
with the MSbP system.

XII. SUMMARY

Only through the perspective of clinical social psychology is it possible to perceive and analyze pathological group processes.

With this new perspective, the "MSbP as a group phenomenon" in the field of autism was examined and presented as an example.

By analyzing it becomes clear that

• MSbP occurs much more frequently than previously assumed.

• Pathological behavior can be publicly carried out within group structures and still remain undetected for decades.

• the distribution of individual motives and actions among different actors within different subgroups has a stabilizing and legitimizing effect.

• The role of the perpetrator in the abuse is not limited to the primary caregivers.

• It is possible that the child could be harmed against the parents' actual will.

1   Need for clinical social psychology

The fact that the MSbP as a group phenomenon in the field of autism could exist within psychology for over

half a century - and remained undiscovered, vividly demonstrates the need for rapid development of a systematically structured clinical social psychology.

XIII. APPENDIX: AUTISM AS VUL-
NERABILITY

Our analytical thinking leads to us breaking things down into their components and trying to fathom the properties of the whole based on its parts. Vygotsky (1993) illustrates the resulting problems using the example of analyzing the properties of water based on the properties of its constituents - hydrogen and oxygen. It becomes clear that the property of water to extinguish fire cannot be explained by the properties of the two constituents that burn (hydrogen) or that make a fire possible in the first place (oxygen).

In the normal development of a child, it is still relatively easy for us to imagine the need for an interaction between child and environment, both social and physical.

The child develops through the interaction of his own maturation processes with the development of social interaction (Vygotsky 1993).

If the child's development is disturbed, we quickly fall back into the analytical division between child and environment. And as a result we look for the reasons for the disturbed development in the child.

Vygotsky (1993) explains this using the example of a blind child whose disorder is not "blindness", but the resulting disruption of social interaction.

In a group of cavemen who only live in their lightless cave, the blind child would not even be perceived as blind.

Only the combination of the child's limitation with the social environment creates the disorder - the disorder of social interaction. And it is only when the social interaction necessary for development is disturbed that development is disturbed.

This disruption of development can in turn lead to disruption of social interaction and so on.

As explained in detail in Schmidt (2015a, 2015b), Schmidt / Ganz (2016), Schmidt / Döhler / Döhler (2017), there are two risks in autistic people that there will be a disruption of conscious social interaction.

1. On the one hand, autistic people lack unconscious group communication.

Second, autistic people have a combination of hypersensitivity and stimulus filter weakness.

Both of these mean that autistic people have a higher risk of fear and stress, which prevent a "relaxed field" (Hassenstein 1987, Eibl-Eibesfeldt 2004) and thus the prerequisites for play and relaxed social communication. This leads to a "disruption of social interaction".

This disorder in turn can lead to a "profound developmental disorder".

Appropriate therapies, such as child-centered approaches, therefore aim to restore social interaction in order to remedy the developmental disturbance. The first step is to create a "relaxed field". In an environment that induces stress and anxiety, the child is unable to communicate and interact, at least in the early stages of development. However, it is precisely the disruption of social communication and interaction that makes these children particularly susceptible to abuse.

"Although it is rare for victims of any age to recognize and report to others that they are being subjected to MBP abuse or neglect, those with genuine mental health or developmental impairments are generally more dependent on their caregivers than their healthy peers, and some have significant communication deficits. Such students are highly vulnerable to victimization and less able to identify and report it (Randall & Parker, 1997)."
[Schreier et al. 2018]

BIBLIOGRAPHY

autismus Deutschland e.V. (2016): Einschätzung des wissenschaftlichen Beirates des Verbandes „Autismus Deutschland e. V." zur „Stellungnahme gegen ABA" des Vereinvorstandes Regionalverband Autismus Mittelfranken e.V. Autismus Deutschland, zuletzt geprüft am 16.05.2016.

autismus Deutschland e.V. (2020): Positionspapier „Zur Notwendigkeit einer autismusspezifischen Frühtherapie". Unter Mitarbeit von Prof. Dr. Dr. Kai Vogeley, Prof. Dr. Matthias Dalferth, Prof. Dr. med. Matthias Dose, Prof. Dr. med. Dipl. theol. Christine M. Freitag, Prof. Dr. phil. Inge Kamp-Becker, Claus Lechmann et al. Online verfügbar unter https://www.autismus.de/fileadmin/RECHT_UND_GESELLSCHA FT/Positionspapier_Fruehtherapie19.05.2020.pdf, zuletzt aktualisiert am 24.09.2020.

autismus Mittelfranken e.V. (2016): Stellungnahme gegen ABA, zuletzt geprüft am 16.05.2016.

Ayoub, Catherine C.; Schreier, Herbert A.; Keller, Carol (2002): Munchausen by proxy: presentations in special education. In: *Child maltreatment* 7 (2), S. 149–159. DOI: 10.1177/1077559502007002007.

Barrett, Stephen (2020): A Critical Look at Defeat Autism Now! and the "DAN! Protocol" | Quackwatch. Online verfügbar unter https://quackwatch.org/consumer-education/nonrecorg/dan/, zuletzt aktualisiert am 24.09.2020, zuletzt geprüft am 24.09.2020.

Bettelheim, Bruno (1967): The Empty Fortress. Infantile Autism and the Birth of Self. The Free Press, New York

Davis, Paul; Murtagh, Una; Glaser, Danya (2019): 40 years of fabricated or induced illness (FII): where next for paediatricians? Paper 1: epidemiology and definition of FII. In: *Archives of disease in childhood* 104 (2), S. 110–114. DOI: 10.1136/archdischild-2017-314319.

Eibl-Eibesfeldt, Irenäus (2004): Die Biologie des menschlichen Verhaltens. Grundriss der Humanethologie. 5. Aufl., genehmigte Sonderausg. Vierkirchen-Pasenbach: Blank-Media.

Feldman, M. D. (1994): Denial in Munchausen syndrome by proxy: the consulting psychiatrist's dilemma. In: *International journal of psychiatry in medicine* 24 (2), S. 121–128. DOI: 10.2190/1B42-9RD9-H1PE-7UVF.

Flaherty, Emalee G.; Macmillan, Harriet L. (2013): Caregiver-fabricated illness in a child: a manifestation of child maltreatment. In: *Pediatrics* 132 (3), S. 590–597. DOI: 10.1542/peds.2013-2045.

Frye, Ellen M.; Feldman, Marc D. (2012): Factitious Disorder by Proxy in Educational Settings: A Review. In: *Educ Psychol Rev* 24 (1), S. 47–61. DOI: 10.1007/s10648-011-9180-9.

Ganz, Andreas; Schmidt, Bernhard J. (2016): Klartext kompakt. Frühkindlicher Autismus: Verstehen = Helfen. 1. Auflage. Norderstedt: Books on Demand (Klartext kompakt, 8).

Hassenstein, Bernhard (1987): Verhaltensbiologie des Kindes. 4., überarb. und erw. Aufl. München: Piper.

Hirvikoski, Tatja; Mittendorfer-Rutz, Ellenor; Boman, Marcus; Larsson, Henrik; Lichtenstein, Paul; Bölte, Sven (2016): Premature mortality in autism spectrum disorder. In: *The British journal of psychiatry : the journal of mental science* 208 (3), S. 232–238. DOI: 10.1192/bjp.bp.114.160192.

Levy, David M. (1950): Maternal Overprotection. 4. Aufl. New York: Columbia University Press.

Majda, Katarzyna; Dudzik, Katarzyna; Jarząbkowska, Angelika; Łakomska, Oliwia (2019): Munchausen syndrome by proxy. Causes, signs and treatment. DOI: 10.5281/zenodo.3408272.

Meadow, Roy (1977): MUNCHAUSEN SYNDROME BY PROXY THE HINTERLAND OF CHILD ABUSE. In: *The Lancet* 310 (8033), S. 343–345. DOI: 10.1016/S0140-6736(77)91497-0.

Pangborn, Jon; Baker, Sidney M. (2005): Autism. Effective biomedical treatments : have we done everyting we can for this child? : individuality in an autism epidemic. Boston DAN! April 2005 ed. Boston

Randall, Pete; Parker, Jon (1997): Factitious Disorder by Proxy and the Abuse of a Child with Autism. In: *Educational Psychology in Practice* 13 (1), S. 39–45. DOI: 10.1080/0266736970130108.

Rimland, Bernard (1964): Infantile Autism. The syndrome and its implications for a neural theory of behavior. (New York: Appleton-Century-Crofts (The Century Psychology Series), 1962).

Schmidt, Bernhard J. (2015a): Autistic and Society - An angry change of perspective. Volume 1: Understanding Autism. Norderstedt: Books on Demand.

- (2015b): Autistic and Society - An angry change of perspective. Volume 2: Support for Autistic? Norderstedt: Books on Demand

- (2016): Autismus. Wenn Händewaschen hilft. 1. Auflage. Norderstedt: Books on Demand.

- (2017a): Autismus. Und vorgetäuschte Hilfe. 1. Auflage. Norderstedt: Books on Demand.

- (2018): BauSÄTZE: Frames - als Be-Deutungs-Rahmen. Beiträge zur Wissens(chafts)-Psychologie. 1. Auflage. Norderstedt: BoD

- (2019): BauSÄTZE: Begriffe - Gedanken - Hypothesen - Theorien II. Beiträge zur Wissens(chafts)-Psychologie. 1. Auflage. Norderstedt: BoD

- (2019b): Autism and the Refrigerator Mother Myth. A Rehabilitation of Bruno Bettelheim. 1. Edition. Norderstedt: BoD – Books on Demand (Contributions to the Psychology of Science, 1).

- (2020): AUTISM - BLAMING THE PARENTS. Research between Dogma and Taboo.: Books on Demand.

Schmidt, Bernhard J.; Döhler, Christiane; Döhler, Deniz (2017): Autism - Sexuality - Relationships. 1. Auflage. Norderstedt: Books on Demand (Contributions to the clinical sozial psychology, 6).

Schmidt, Bernhard J.; Ganz, Andreas (2016): Plaintext compact. The Asperger Syndrom. Not only for Psychotherapists. 1. Edition. Norderstedt: Books on Demand.

- (2017): Symbiotischer Narzissmus als Gruppenphänomen. Norderstedt: Books on Demand (Beiträge zur klinischen Sozialpsychologie, 5).

Schreier, H. A. (2000): Factitious disorder by proxy in which the presenting problem is behavioral or psychiatric. In: *Journal of the American Academy of Child and Adolescent Psychiatry* 39 (5), S. 668–670. DOI: 10.1097/00004583-200005000-00022.

Schreier, Herbert A.; Bursch, Brenda (2018): Munchausen by Proxy in Educational and Mental Health Settings. In: *ADVISOR*, S. 61–65. Online verfügbar unter http://ican4kids.org/Nexus/Claudia%20Wang.pdf.

Sheridan, Mary S. (2003): The deceit continues: an updated literature review of Munchausen Syndrome by Proxy. In: *Child Abuse & Neglect* 27 (4), S. 431–451. DOI: 10.1016/S0145-2134(03)00030-9.

Tinbergen, Nikolaas (1974): Ethology and Stress Diseases. In: *Science* 185 (4145), S. 20–27. Online verfügbar unter http://www.jstor.org/stable/1738611.

Tinbergen, Niko; Tinbergen, Elisabeth A. (1983): "Autistic" children. New hope for a cure. London: Allen & Unwin.

Vllasaliu, Leonora (2016): Autismus-Spektrum-Störungen im Kindes-, Jugend- und Erwachsenenalter. Interdisziplinäre S3-Leitlinie der DGKJP und der DGPPN sowie der beteiligten Fachgesellschaften, Berufsverbände und Patientenorganisationen, zuletzt geprüft am 24.09.2020.

Vygotsky, Lev Semenovič (1993): The fundamentals of defectology. . New York: Plenum Press (The collected works of L. S. Vygotsky, 2).

Vygotsky, Lev Semenovič; Bruner, Jerome S. (1987): Problems of general psychology. Including the volume "Thinking and speech". New York: Plenum Press (The collected works of L. S. Vygotsky, 1).

Vygotsky, Lev Semenovič; Cole, Michael (1981): Mind in society. The development of higher psychological processes. [Nachdr.]. Cambridge, Mass.: Harvard Univ. Press.

Vygotsky, Lev Semenovič; Ratner, Carl (1998): Child psychology. New York: Plenum Press (The collected works of L. S. Vygotsky, 5).

Warner, J. O.; Hathaway, M. J. (1984): Allergic form of Meadow's syndrome (Munchausen by proxy). In: *Archives of disease in childhood* 59 (2), S. 151–156. DOI: 10.1136/adc.59.2.151.

Waterhouse, Lynn H. (Hg.) (2013): Rethinking autism. Variation and complexity. 1st ed. London, Waltham, MA: Academic Press.

Waterhouse, Lynn; London, Eric; Gillberg, Christopher (2016): ASD Validity. In: *Rev J Autism Dev Disord* 3 (4), S. 302–329. DOI: 10.1007/s40489-016-0085-x.

West, Charles Kenyon (1981): The social and psychological distortion of information. Charles K. West. Chicago: Nelson-Hall.

Wetherell, Margaret (Hg.) (1996): Identities, groups and social issues. London: SAGE (Social psychology, 3).

Wing, John K. (Hg.) (1966): Early childhood autism. Clinical, educational and social aspects. 1. ed. Oxford: Pergamon Pr.

Wing, L. (Hg.) (1976): Early childhood autism. Clinical, educational and social aspects. 2nd ed. Oxford, New York, Oxford: Pergamon Press (Pergamon international library of science, technology, engineering and social studies).

Zarankiewicz, Natalia; Zielińska, Martyna; Kosz, Katarzyna; Kuchnicka, Aleksandra; Siedlecki, Wojciech; Książek, Katarzyna; Mojsym Korybska, Sylwia (2019): The art of cheating medical staff - Munchausen Syndrome by Proxy. DOI: 10.5281/zenodo.3358650.